GESTATIONAL DIABETES FOOD LIST

The Complete Ingredient list and Food to Avoid for Gestational Diabetes

Harley W. Norman

Copyright © 2024 by Harley W. Norman

All rights reserved

No part of this publication may be reproduced, stored in a retrieval system. or transmitted. in and form or by any means, electronic, mechanical, photocopying, recording, or otherwise, without the prior written permission of the author. The information in this eBook is true and complete to the best

of our knowledge. All recommendations are made without guarantee on the part of the author or publisher. The author and publisher disclaim any liability in connection with the use of this information.

Table of Contents

Introduction to Gestational Diabetes 6

    Understanding Gestational Diabetes 9

    Impact on Pregnancy and Baby 13

    The Role of Diet in Managing Gestational Diabetes 16

Nutritional Foundations for Gestational Diabetes 20

    Macronutrients: Carbohydrates, Proteins, and Fats 20

    Micronutrients and Their Importance 25

Safe and Beneficial Foods for Gestational Diabetes 29

    Whole Grains and Why They Matter 29

    Vegetables: A Rainbow on Your Plate 34

    Fruits: Understanding Glycemic Index 38

    Proteins: Animal vs. Plant-Based Sources 42

    Fats: Identifying Healthy Fats 48

    Dairy: Options and Alternatives 53

    Snacks: Healthy Choices to Keep You Going 59

Foods to Limit or Avoid 64

    High Glycemic Index Fruits and Vegetables 64

    Processed and Junk Foods 69

    Sugary Beverages and Sweets 73

    Fatty Meats and High-Fat Dairy Products 77

    Alcohol and Caffeine 80

Reading Food Labels 83

    Understanding Carbohydrate Counts 83

    Identifying Added Sugars 87

    Recognizing Healthy Fats 90

Meal Planning and Preparation 93

    Sample Meal Plans 93

    Shopping List Essentials 96

    Meal Prep Tips for Busy Expectant Mothers 99

Eating Out and Social Events 102

    Tips for Restaurant Dining 102

    Navigating Social Gatherings 105

    Alcohol Alternatives and Mocktails 108

Monitoring Blood Sugar Levels 111

    The Importance of Monitoring 111

    How Food Affects Blood Sugar 114

    Adjusting Your Diet Based on Blood Sugar Readings 117

Exercise and Physical Activity 120

    Safe Exercises During Pregnancy 120

The Impact of Physical Activity on Gestational Diabetes 124

Conclusion 127

Introduction to Gestational Diabetes

In the town of Evergreen, nestled between rolling hills and vibrant meadows, lived a woman named Ella. Ella, a nutritionist by profession and a storyteller at heart, had a passion for weaving tales that not only entertained but also educated. Her latest project was inspired by a close friend, Lily, who was navigating the complexities of gestational diabetes. Witnessing Lily's struggles and triumphs became the catalyst for Ella's most heartfelt work yet: "The Wholesome Journey: A Gestational Diabetes Food Odyssey."

The story opens on a crisp autumn morning, with our heroine, Lila, facing the challenge of gestational diabetes. Feeling overwhelmed by the diagnosis, Lila's world turns gray, her joy overshadowed by fear and uncertainty. Enter a wise and whimsical owl, Ollie, who overhears Lila's concerns. Ollie, with his vast knowledge and gentle demeanor, offers to guide Lila through the enchanting world of food, promising a journey that would illuminate her path to wellness.

As Lila and Ollie embark on their odyssey, readers are whisked away to magical lands where foods speak, sharing their secrets and powers. They visit the Whispering Wheat Fields, where whole grains teach Lila about the importance of complex carbohydrates for maintaining stable blood sugar levels. In the Verdant Vegetable Valley, vibrant vegetables showcase their low glycemic indices and rich nutrients, empowering Lila to paint her plate with a rainbow of health.

The duo's adventures also lead them to the Dairy Dell, where Lila learns to choose high-quality, low-fat dairy options, and the Protein Peaks, where both plant and animal proteins share the spotlight, emphasizing their essential role in a balanced diet. But not all is light and easy; the duo must navigate the Treacherous Treats Trap, where processed foods and sugary snares lie in wait, teaching Lila the value of moderation and the art of making wise choices.

Each chapter closes with practical tips, easy recipes, and motivational quotes, transforming Lila's journey into a tangible guide for readers. Ella's storytelling magic weaves complex nutritional guidelines into an engaging narrative, making "The Wholesome Journey" not just a book, but a companion for expectant mothers facing gestational diabetes.

Why should one buy this book? Beyond its enchanting story, it stands as a beacon of hope, a testament to the power of knowledge and the strength of the human spirit. It demystifies gestational diabetes, making management through diet feel not only achievable but also enjoyable. Ella, through Lila's journey, assures her readers that with the right guidance, they can turn challenges into victories, fear into confidence, and food into medicine.

As the story of Lila concludes, readers find her not at the end of a journey but at the beginning of a new chapter, equipped with knowledge, empowered by choice, and enveloped in the warmth of Ollie's wisdom. "The Wholesome Journey: A Gestational Diabetes Food Odyssey" is more than a book; it's a lifeline, a friend, and a guide, urging its readers to embrace their journey with gestational diabetes, not with fear, but with courage, knowledge, and a spoonful of joy.

Understanding Gestational Diabetes

Gestational diabetes is a condition that occurs when blood sugar levels become elevated during pregnancy and can impact both the mother and baby's health. Unlike other forms of diabetes, gestational diabetes is usually temporary, resolving after the birth of the baby, but it requires careful management to ensure the well-being of both mother and child. The key to managing gestational diabetes effectively lies in understanding how different foods influence blood sugar levels and how to balance these within a nutritious pregnancy diet.

The cornerstone of managing gestational diabetes is a diet that prioritizes blood sugar control. This involves choosing foods with a low to moderate glycemic index (GI), which refers to how quickly foods raise blood sugar levels. Foods with a lower GI release glucose slowly and steadily, preventing the spikes in blood sugar that can be harmful during pregnancy. Whole grains, such as brown rice, quinoa, and whole wheat bread, are excellent choices as they are digested more slowly, providing steady energy and keeping blood sugar levels stable.

Vegetables are another crucial component of a gestational diabetes-friendly diet. Rich in fiber, vitamins, and minerals, they have a minimal impact on blood sugar levels. Non-starchy vegetables like leafy greens, peppers, and broccoli are particularly beneficial as they provide essential nutrients without contributing to blood sugar spikes. In contrast, starchy vegetables such as potatoes and corn should be consumed in moderation due to their higher carbohydrate content.

Fruits, while nutritious, contain natural sugars and can affect blood sugar levels. Choosing fruits with a lower glycemic index, such as berries, apples, and pears, can help manage blood sugar. Portion control is also important; pairing fruits with a protein or healthy fat can help stabilize blood sugar levels. For example, an apple with a handful of almonds offers a balanced snack by combining the fruit's carbohydrates with the almonds' healthy fats and protein.

Proteins are a vital part of the diet and have little to no impact on blood sugar levels, making them a safe choice for women with gestational diabetes. Lean protein sources, such as chicken, fish, tofu, and legumes, provide the necessary nutrients without adding excessive calories or fats. Including a source of protein at each meal can help maintain muscle mass and keep hunger at bay.

Dairy products offer calcium and protein but can vary in their carbohydrate content. Choosing lower-fat and lower-sugar dairy options, such as plain Greek yogurt or skim milk, can provide the benefits of dairy without elevating blood sugar levels excessively.

Fats are essential for the body's overall health but choosing the right type of fat is key. Unsaturated fats found in avocados, nuts, seeds, and olive oil are healthier choices, providing essential fatty acids without negatively impacting blood sugar levels.

Understanding how to read food labels is an important skill for managing gestational diabetes. Labels provide information on the amount of carbohydrates, sugars, protein, and fat in foods, helping women make informed choices about what to include in their diet.

Meal planning and preparation play a significant role in managing gestational diabetes. Planning meals ahead of time can ensure that the diet remains balanced and blood sugar levels stay controlled. Preparing meals and snacks at home allows for better control over ingredients and portion sizes, essential aspects of gestational diabetes management.

In summary, managing gestational diabetes through diet involves choosing low-glycemic foods, focusing on fiber-rich vegetables, incorporating lean proteins, selecting low-sugar fruits, opting for healthy fats, and understanding food labels for better meal planning. These dietary strategies not only help control blood sugar levels during pregnancy but also contribute to overall health and well-being for both mother and baby.

Impact on Pregnancy and Baby

Gestational diabetes, a condition characterized by elevated blood glucose levels during pregnancy, poses unique challenges and risks to both the expecting mother and her baby. It primarily emerges in the second or third trimester when pregnancy hormones interfere with the body's ability to use insulin effectively, leading to insulin resistance. Without proper management, gestational diabetes can have significant impacts on pregnancy and the baby, making a well-considered diet an essential tool for control and prevention of complications.

For the pregnant woman, gestational diabetes increases the risk of developing high blood pressure and preeclampsia, a serious condition that can threaten the lives of both mother and baby. It also raises the likelihood of requiring a Cesarean section due to the baby's increased size, a direct result of high blood sugar levels. Moreover, women with gestational diabetes are more likely to develop type 2 diabetes later in life, making it imperative to adhere to a healthy diet during pregnancy to minimize these risks.

The baby, too, faces challenges when the mother has uncontrolled gestational diabetes. High blood sugar levels in the mother lead to high blood sugar levels in the baby, prompting the baby's pancreas to produce extra insulin. This can cause the baby to grow excessively large (a condition known as macrosomia), complicating delivery and increasing the risk of injury during birth. Babies born to mothers with gestational diabetes are also at a higher risk of developing low blood sugar (hypoglycemia) shortly after birth, which can lead to seizures if not treated promptly. Furthermore, these babies have a higher chance of becoming overweight and developing type 2 diabetes as they grow older.

Incorporating a gestational diabetes-friendly food list into daily meals can significantly mitigate these risks. Such a diet emphasizes the importance of balancing macronutrients—carbohydrates, proteins, and fats—to maintain stable blood sugar levels. Foods low in simple sugars and high in complex carbohydrates and fiber, such as whole grains, vegetables, and certain fruits, are encouraged because they have a more gradual effect on blood sugar. Lean protein sources and healthy fats are also pivotal, supporting maternal and fetal health without exacerbating insulin resistance.

Equally important is the avoidance of foods that can spike blood sugar levels, including processed foods, sugary beverages, and sweets. By focusing on nutrient-dense foods and practicing portion control, expecting mothers can help ensure their own health and their baby's well-being. Additionally, frequent, small meals and snacks can help prevent the blood sugar peaks and valleys that are particularly detrimental during pregnancy.

Ultimately, the impact of gestational diabetes on pregnancy and the baby underscores the importance of dietary management as part of a comprehensive approach to care. Through careful food choices, based on a gestational diabetes food list, expectant mothers can help protect their health and set the stage for a healthy start for their babies. This proactive nutritional strategy not only addresses the immediate concerns associated with gestational diabetes but also contributes to long-term health benefits for both mother and child, making it a critical aspect of gestational diabetes management.

The Role of Diet in Managing Gestational Diabetes

Managing gestational diabetes is a critical aspect of prenatal care, ensuring both maternal and fetal health. The cornerstone of this management is diet, which plays a pivotal role in controlling blood glucose levels to prevent complications. A carefully curated gestational diabetes food list is not just a tool; it's a roadmap to a healthier pregnancy.

Gestational diabetes occurs when the body cannot effectively use insulin during pregnancy, leading to elevated blood glucose levels. Since insulin does not cross the placenta but glucose does, managing dietary intake of carbohydrates—the primary macronutrient affecting blood glucose—is paramount. This is where the gestational diabetes food list comes into play, emphasizing foods that help maintain steady blood glucose levels.

Whole grains are a staple in this dietary approach. Unlike their refined counterparts, whole grains are rich in fiber, which slows the absorption of sugar into the bloodstream. Foods like quinoa, brown rice, and oats are not only nutritious but also versatile, easily incorporated into daily meals.

Vegetables, particularly non-starchy ones such as leafy greens, bell peppers, and broccoli, are another cornerstone. They offer essential nutrients and fiber, supporting overall health while helping to keep blood sugar levels in check. The list encourages a "rainbow on your plate" approach, ensuring a wide array of vitamins and minerals.

Fruits, while nutritious, require careful consideration due to their natural sugars. The focus is on those with a lower glycemic index, which have a more gradual effect on blood sugar levels. Berries, apples, and pears, enjoyed in moderation and paired with a protein or fat, can be part of a balanced diet.

Proteins are critical for fetal development and help stabilize blood glucose by slowing digestion. The list highlights lean sources, both animal-based (like chicken breast and fish) and plant-based (such as lentils and chickpeas), to provide variety and essential nutrients without excess fat.

Healthy fats from sources like avocados, nuts, and olive oil are included for their ability to provide satiety and support cell growth without spiking blood sugar. These fats are crucial for absorbing certain vitamins and providing a steady energy source.

Dairy products selected are those low in sugar yet high in calcium and protein, such as Greek yogurt and cottage cheese. These choices support bone health while fitting into a gestational diabetes-friendly diet.

Beyond specific foods, the list advocates for balance and portion control, emphasizing the importance of spreading carbohydrate intake evenly throughout the day to prevent spikes in blood glucose levels. It also suggests pairing carbohydrates with proteins or fats to further stabilize blood sugar.

Meal planning and preparation become vital tools, enabling expectant mothers to have nutritious options readily available. This approach prevents impulsive eating decisions that might lead to suboptimal food choices.

Lastly, the role of diet in managing gestational diabetes extends beyond the pregnancy. Adopting these dietary guidelines can pave the way for a healthier postpartum period and potentially mitigate the risk of developing type 2 diabetes later in life. This food list, therefore, is more than a temporary regimen; it's a step towards lasting health for both mother and child.

In summary, the gestational diabetes food list is a meticulously designed guide that supports blood glucose management through a balanced, nutrient-rich diet. It empowers expectant mothers to make informed food choices, ensuring the well-being of both themselves and their babies. Through education and adherence to this dietary framework, managing gestational diabetes becomes an attainable goal, marked by informed choices and healthier outcomes.

Nutritional Foundations for Gestational Diabetes

Macronutrients: Carbohydrates, Proteins, and Fats

Understanding macronutrients—carbohydrates, proteins, and fats—is foundational for managing gestational diabetes effectively. These nutritional building blocks play distinct roles in the body, especially important during pregnancy, when both the mother's and the developing baby's health are at stake. A gestational diabetes food list centered around the mindful selection and balance of these macronutrients can help control blood glucose levels while ensuring both mother and baby receive the nutrients they need.

The Importance of Carbohydrate Counting

Carbohydrates are the primary energy source for the body and have the most immediate impact on blood glucose levels. Managing gestational diabetes requires careful attention to both the quantity and type of carbohydrates consumed. Carbohydrate counting is a method used to monitor the amount of carbohydrates eaten at meals and snacks. It involves keeping track of the number of carbohydrate grams in the foods consumed, aiming to spread carbohydrate intake evenly throughout the day to avoid spikes in blood glucose levels.

Whole grains, fruits, vegetables, and legumes are preferred carbohydrate sources because they are rich in fiber, which slows glucose absorption into the bloodstream, preventing sudden spikes in blood sugar. For example, opting for a serving of quinoa or brown rice instead of white rice can make a significant difference in blood glucose control. Understanding and implementing carbohydrate counting allows for flexibility and precision in managing gestational diabetes, making it a critical aspect of dietary planning.

Selecting Healthy Proteins

Proteins are crucial for the growth and repair of body tissues, and they play a vital role in the development of the fetus. Unlike carbohydrates, proteins have a minimal impact on blood glucose levels, making them an essential component of a gestational diabetes diet. Healthy protein choices include lean meats, poultry, fish, eggs, dairy products, beans, lentils, and tofu. These proteins provide the necessary amino acids for fetal development without contributing to excessive blood glucose fluctuations.

Incorporating a variety of protein sources in the diet not only supports maternal and fetal health but also aids in feeling satiated, which can help control overall calorie intake and support healthy pregnancy weight gain. For instance, adding a portion of grilled chicken breast to a salad or including a serving of lentils in a soup can boost protein intake, contributing to a balanced meal plan.

Choosing the Right Fats

Fats are essential for the absorption of certain vitamins and are a critical energy source for the body. However, not all fats are created equal, especially in the context of gestational diabetes. Unsaturated fats, found in foods like avocados, nuts, seeds, and olive oil, are beneficial for heart health and should be the primary fat sources in the diet. These fats can help improve blood cholesterol levels and offer anti-inflammatory properties, which are beneficial during pregnancy.

In contrast, saturated fats, found in red meat and full-fat dairy products, and trans fats, found in processed foods, should be limited. These fats can contribute to heart disease and may negatively impact glucose metabolism. Replacing unhealthy fats with healthier options, such as cooking with olive oil instead of butter or choosing lean cuts of meat, can support overall health and gestational diabetes management.

Integrating Macronutrients into the Gestational Diabetes Food List

A gestational diabetes food list incorporating the right balance of carbohydrates, proteins, and fats is crucial for managing blood glucose levels and supporting a healthy pregnancy. This list emphasizes whole, nutrient-dense foods that provide energy and support fetal development while minimizing the risk of gestational diabetes complications.

Balancing these macronutrients involves thoughtful meal planning. For example, a breakfast might include a small portion of whole-grain toast with avocado and a side of scrambled eggs, providing a balanced mix of carbohydrates, healthy fats, and proteins. Snacks might consist of Greek yogurt with a handful of berries, offering protein, carbohydrates, and a rich source of vitamins and antioxidants.

By focusing on the quality and balance of macronutrients, expectant mothers can manage gestational diabetes more effectively, ensuring optimal health for themselves and their babies. This approach to diet underscores the importance of nutrition education in the management of gestational diabetes, empowering women to make informed choices about their eating habits during this critical time.

Micronutrients and Their Importance

In the landscape of managing gestational diabetes, while macronutrients often steal the spotlight for their direct impact on blood sugar levels, the nuanced role of micronutrients cannot be overstated. Vitamins and minerals, though required in smaller quantities, are pivotal in ensuring both maternal well-being and fetal development. Their importance in the nutritional foundation for gestational diabetes is critical, as they influence everything from blood sugar control to the body's response to insulin.

Vitamins to Focus On

Vitamin D is essential for calcium absorption, bone health, and immune function. Research suggests it also plays a role in glucose metabolism, making it a vital component for managing gestational diabetes. Sources include fortified foods, egg yolks, and safe sun exposure.

Vitamin C enhances iron absorption and is crucial for tissue repair and growth. Its antioxidant properties also protect cells from damage. Citrus fruits, strawberries, bell peppers, and leafy greens are excellent sources.

B Vitamins, particularly folic acid (B9), B6, and B12, support fetal brain development and reduce the risk of neural tube defects. They also aid in energy metabolism. Lean meats, legumes, nuts, and fortified cereals are rich in B vitamins.

Vitamin E is an antioxidant that helps protect cells from oxidative stress. While excessive amounts can be harmful, adequate intake through diet is beneficial for both mother and child. Almonds, spinach, and sweet potatoes are good sources.

Minerals to Focus On

Calcium is crucial for building strong bones and teeth in the fetus and maintaining the mother's bone density. It also plays a role in nerve transmission and muscle function. Dairy products, fortified plant milks, and green leafy vegetables are high in calcium.

Iron supports the increased blood volume during pregnancy and is vital for oxygen transport and cell growth. Iron deficiency is a common issue in pregnancy and can lead to anemia. Lean meats, legumes, and fortified grains are key sources.

Magnesium helps regulate blood sugar levels and supports over 300 enzymatic reactions, including those important for protein synthesis and blood pressure regulation. Nuts, seeds, and whole grains are excellent sources.

Zinc is essential for DNA synthesis, cell division, and proper immune function. It also supports normal growth and development during pregnancy. Foods rich in zinc include meat, dairy products, nuts, and whole grains.

Hydration and Gestational Diabetes

Hydration plays a non-negotiable role in the management of gestational diabetes. Adequate fluid intake helps in the regulation of blood sugar levels, aids in digestion, and prevents constipation—a common issue in pregnancy. Moreover, staying hydrated helps reduce the risk of urinary tract infections, which pregnant women are more prone to.

Water is the best choice for staying hydrated. It's calorie-free, sugar-free, and readily available. Pregnant women should aim for at least 8-12 cups of fluids daily, with needs increasing in hot weather or with physical activity. While water should make up the majority of fluid intake, other beverages like milk and small amounts of 100% fruit juice can contribute to hydration. However, it's crucial to avoid sugary drinks and those with artificial sweeteners, as they can impact blood sugar control.

In conclusion, the emphasis on micronutrients and hydration within the nutritional foundations for managing gestational diabetes highlights the holistic approach needed for optimal health outcomes. A gestational diabetes food list that incorporates a wide variety of vitamins and minerals, along with a focus on hydration, supports not just the management of blood sugar levels but the overall health of the mother and the developing fetus. This comprehensive approach ensures that both immediate and long-term health goals are addressed, paving the way for a healthy pregnancy and beyond.

Safe and Beneficial Foods for Gestational Diabetes

Whole Grains and Why They Matter

Whole grains are a fundamental component of a gestational diabetes diet, offering a powerhouse of nutrients along with the necessary fiber to help manage blood sugar levels effectively. Their inclusion in a gestational diabetes food list is backed by substantial evidence highlighting their benefits for both maternal health and fetal development.

The table below details various whole grain options and elucidates why they matter in the context of managing gestational diabetes.

Whole Grain Options	Why They Matter
Quinoa	Quinoa is a complete protein, containing all nine essential amino acids, which is rare for plant foods. It's also high in fiber, which can help manage blood sugar levels by slowing down the absorption of carbohydrates. Additionally, quinoa provides iron,

Whole Grain Options	Why They Matter
	magnesium, and B vitamins, supporting overall maternal health.
Brown Rice	Unlike white rice, brown rice retains its outer bran layer, making it a good source of fiber, vitamins, and minerals like magnesium, which is important for blood sugar regulation. Its lower glycemic index compared to white rice makes it a safer option for managing blood sugar levels.
Whole Oatmeal	Oats are particularly high in beta-glucan, a type of soluble fiber that helps control blood sugar by delaying stomach emptying and the absorption of glucose into the bloodstream. They're also a great source of magnesium, which plays a role in insulin regulation.
Barley	Barley has a low glycemic index and is rich in beta-glucan fiber, helping to slow glucose absorption. It's beneficial for heart health and blood sugar control, making it an excellent choice for women managing

Whole Grain Options	Why They Matter
	gestational diabetes.
Whole Grain Bread	Bread made from whole grains rather than refined flour contains more nutrients and fiber. This fiber helps moderate blood sugar spikes after meals, making whole grain bread a better choice for maintaining steady glucose levels.
Bulgur Wheat	Bulgur is a whole grain that's partially precooked, making it a quick and easy option for meals. It's high in fiber and has a low glycemic index, which can help in managing blood sugar levels more effectively. Plus, it offers a good dose of B vitamins and minerals like iron and magnesium.
Farro	Farro is an ancient grain with a chewy texture and nutty flavor, high in fiber, antioxidants, and B vitamins. It has a lower glycemic index, which is beneficial for blood sugar control in gestational diabetes.
Freekeh	Freekeh is a young green wheat that's harvested while still tender, then roasted and cracked. This process retains more nutrients, including fiber and protein,

Whole Grain Options	Why They Matter
	than mature wheat, helping to support blood sugar management.

Whole grains matter in the context of gestational diabetes for several reasons. They provide a sustained energy source, preventing rapid spikes in blood glucose that can occur with the consumption of refined carbohydrates. The high fiber content in whole grains slows down the digestion and absorption of sugar, offering a steadier source of glucose for the body's needs. This is crucial for maintaining optimal blood sugar levels throughout pregnancy.

Furthermore, the rich nutrient profile of whole grains, including vitamins, minerals, and antioxidants, supports overall pregnancy health. These nutrients contribute to fetal development, maternal energy levels, and the prevention of pregnancy-related complications. Incorporating a variety of whole grains into the diet ensures that these benefits are maximized, promoting both maternal and fetal well-being during a time when nutrition is paramount.

In sum, whole grains are an essential element of a gestational diabetes food list, offering broad health benefits beyond just blood sugar management. They provide vital nutrients for pregnancy health, making them an indispensable part of a balanced and nutritious diet for expectant mothers managing gestational diabetes.

Vegetables: A Rainbow on Your Plate

Creating a colorful plate with a variety of vegetables is not just visually appealing; it's a healthful approach to eating, especially important in managing gestational diabetes.

Vegetables, with their low glycemic index and rich nutrient profile, play a pivotal role in stabilizing blood sugar while providing essential vitamins and minerals for both mother and baby.

Color	Vegetables	Benefits	Serving Ideas
Green	Spinach, Broccoli, Kale	Rich in iron, calcium, and folate. Green vegetables are also high in fiber, which helps control blood sugar levels.	Add spinach to smoothies, stir-fry broccoli, or make kale chips.
Red	Tomatoes, Red Peppers	High in antioxidants like lycopene and vitamin C, which can help with iron absorption and support immune function.	Slice tomatoes for salads, roast red peppers for a rich flavor.

Color	Vegetables	Benefits	Serving Ideas
Yellow	Summer Squash, Corn	Contains antioxidants such as lutein, which supports eye health. Note: Corn should be consumed in moderation due to its higher glycemic index.	Grill summer squash or add corn to a vegetable medley (in moderation).
Orange	Carrots, Pumpkin	Rich in beta-carotene, which is converted to vitamin A in the body, supporting vision and immune function.	Snack on raw carrots or use pumpkin in soups.
Purple	Eggplant, Red Cabbage	Contains anthocyanins, powerful antioxidants that may help reduce inflammation and improve heart health.	Bake eggplant slices or add shredded red cabbage to salads for a colorful crunch.
White	Cauliflower, Mushrooms	Offers a variety of nutrients such as choline in cauliflower, which is important for brain health, and selenium in mushrooms.	Roast cauliflower florets or sauté mushrooms as a side.

Color	Vegetables	Benefits	Serving Ideas
		mushrooms, antioxidant.	an

Vegetable Preparation Tips for Gestational Diabetes:

- **Choose Fresh or Frozen:** Fresh vegetables are optimal, but frozen varieties without added sauces or sugars are a convenient and nutritious alternative.
- **Mind the Cooking Method:** Steaming, roasting, or grilling vegetables enhances their flavor without adding unhealthy fats or extra calories.
- **Portion Control:** Even with vegetables, it's important to be mindful of portions, especially for starchy vegetables like corn and potatoes.
- **Incorporate Variety:** Eating a wide range of vegetables ensures a broad intake of different nutrients beneficial for pregnancy.

Incorporating a "rainbow on your plate" is a delightful and healthful way to manage gestational diabetes. This colorful array of vegetables not only makes meals more enjoyable but also ensures that you're getting a wide range of nutrients essential for the health of both mother and baby. By following the serving ideas and preparation tips outlined in the table, you can easily add a variety of nutritious vegetables to your diet, keeping your gestational diabetes in check while supporting overall well-being during pregnancy.

Fruits: Understanding Glycemic Index

The glycemic index (GI) is a crucial tool for managing gestational diabetes, providing a measure of how quickly foods raise blood glucose levels. Fruits, while an essential part of a balanced diet due to their vitamins, minerals, and fiber content, vary significantly in their GI scores. Understanding these variations helps in selecting fruits that contribute to a stable blood sugar level, which is vital for both maternal and fetal health during gestational diabetes.

The table below lists common fruits with their glycemic index values, offering a practical guide for incorporating these nutritious options into a gestational diabetes food list.

Fruit	Glycemic Index (GI)	Serving Size	Notes
Cherries	Low (22)	1 cup (120g)	Rich in antioxidants, cherries have a low GI, making them a good choice for snacking.
Grapefruit	Low (25)	½ medium	This citrus fruit can help control blood sugar, but check with your doctor if on medication.

Fruit	Glycemic Index (GI)	Serving Size	Notes
Apples	Low to Medium (36)	1 small (150g)	Apples are high in fiber and vitamin C, offering a slow release of sugars.
Pears	Low to Medium (38)	1 small (150g)	With their high fiber content, pears are excellent for blood sugar control.
Plums	Low to Medium (40)	1 medium (65g)	Low GI and rich in antioxidants; dried plums (prunes) are higher in GI.
Oranges	Medium (43)	1 medium (130g)	Oranges provide vitamin C and fiber. Peel and eat rather than juice to retain fiber.
Peaches	Medium (42)	1 medium (150g)	Juicy and flavorful, peaches offer a moderate GI and good hydration.
Grapes	Medium (49)	1 cup (150g)	Grapes are higher in sugar; moderation is key.
Kiwifruit	Medium (50)	1 large (120g)	High in vitamin C and fiber, kiwifruits are a nutrient-dense choice.

Fruit	Glycemic Index (GI)	Serving Size	Notes
Banana	Medium to High (51)	1 medium (120g)	Ripe bananas are higher in GI. opt for slightly green bananas for a lower GI.
Watermelon	High (76)	1 cup (150g)	Due to its high GI, watermelon should be consumed in moderation and paired with a protein.
Pineapple	High (59)	1 cup (150g)	Pineapple is higher on the GI scale and should be eaten in small amounts.

Understanding Food Labels for Fruit Selection

When selecting fruits, especially packaged ones, understanding food labels can further aid in managing gestational diabetes. Look for:

- **Total Carbohydrates**: This includes sugars, complex carbohydrates, and fiber. Aim for fruits higher in fiber as it slows glucose absorption.
- **Sugars**: Natural sugars are present in fruits, but it's essential to differentiate these from added sugars in processed fruit products.

- **Serving Size**: Portion control is crucial. Even low-GI fruits can lead to high sugar intake if consumed in large quantities.
- **Added Ingredients**: Avoid fruits with added sugars or syrups. opt for fresh, frozen, or canned fruits in water or their own juice.

By incorporating fruits based on their glycemic index and understanding food labels, individuals with gestational diabetes can enjoy the benefits of these nutritious foods while maintaining optimal blood glucose levels. This approach allows for a varied and enjoyable diet that supports both the health of the mother and the developing fetus.

Proteins: Animal vs. Plant-Based Sources

In managing gestational diabetes, protein plays a crucial role. It's vital for the growth and repair of tissues, plays a part in maintaining blood sugar levels, and can make meals more satisfying, which is particularly important to help manage hunger and blood sugar. When constructing a gestational diabetes-friendly food list, understanding the difference between animal and plant-based protein sources, as well as how to read food labels for these items, is key.

Here's a detailed table comparing animal versus plant-based protein sources, including aspects like typical protein content, additional nutritional benefits, and considerations for gestational diabetes. This comparison not only illuminates the variety available but also highlights how different sources can fit into a gestational diabetes diet.

Protein Source	Type	Typical Protein Content	Other Nutritional Benefits	Considerations for Gestational Diabetes	Reading Food Labels

Protein Source	Type	Typical Protein Content	Other Nutritional Benefits	Considerations for Gestational Diabetes	Reading Food Labels
Chicken breast (cooked)	Animal	31g per 100g	Low in fat (if skinless), contains B vitamins and selenium	Lean option with minimal impact on blood sugar	Look for "skinless" for lower fat options; avoid those prepared with sugary marinades or sauces
Salmon (cooked)	Animal	25g per 100g	High in omega-3 fatty acids, vitamins D and B12	Offers essential fats beneficial for fetal development; low in mercury	opt for wild-caught when possible; check for added sugars or salt in canned versions
Eggs	Animal	6g per large egg	Contains choline, which is	Versatile and can be added to various	Check for added sugar or

Protein Source	Type	Typical Protein Content	Other Nutritional Benefits	Considerations for Gestational Diabetes	Reading Food Labels
			essential for fetal brain development	dishes; monitor for added ingredients in processed egg products	carbohydrates in flavored or processed egg products
					Look for no added sugars or unnecessary additives; sodium content can be high in canned versions
Lentils (cooked)	Plant	9g per 100g	High in fiber, iron, and folate	Helps stabilize blood sugar due to high fiber content	
Quinoa (cooked)	Plant	4g per 100g	Complete protein, high in fiber, magnesium,	Good carbohydrate choice for blood sugar control; can be	Ensure there are no added flavors or sugars; choose

Protein Source	Type	Typical Protein Content	Other Nutritional Benefits	Considerations for Gestational Diabetes	Reading Food Labels
			and iron	a protein and grain in meals	whole grain
Tofu (firm)	Plant	8g per 100g	Contains iron, calcium, and magnesium	Low-calorie, low-carbohydrate source of protein; versatile in recipes	Check for added sugars in flavored varieties; opt for calcium-set tofu for an extra calcium boost
Almonds	Plant	21g per 100g	High in vitamin E, magnesium, and healthy fats	Nutrient-dense snack; mindful of portion sizes due to high calories	Look for raw or dry-roasted without added sugars or excessive salt

Protein Source	Type	Typical Protein Content	Other Nutritional Benefits	Considerations for Gestational Diabetes	Reading Food Labels
Greek yogurt (low-fat)	Animal	10g per 100g	High in calcium, probiotics, and vitamin B12	Balances blood sugar levels; opt for low-fat or non-fat options	Choose plain varieties to avoid added sugars; check carbohydrate content

When incorporating protein into a gestational diabetes diet, it's important to balance both animal and plant-based sources to ensure a wide range of nutrients while managing blood sugar levels. Reading food labels is crucial; look for proteins that are low in saturated fats, free from added sugars, and without unnecessary additives.

For animal proteins, choosing lean cuts and low-fat options can help manage calorie and fat intake. Meanwhile, plant-based proteins often offer the added benefit of fiber, which can assist in blood sugar regulation, but it's essential to be mindful of portion sizes and preparation methods to maintain blood sugar control.

This table serves as a guide to making informed protein choices within a gestational diabetes diet, highlighting the diversity of options available and the considerations needed to optimize health and wellness for both mother and baby.

Fats: Identifying Healthy Fats

When managing gestational diabetes, understanding and choosing the right types of fats can play a significant role in both controlling blood glucose levels and supporting overall pregnancy health. Healthy fats are crucial for fetal development, particularly in the development of the brain and eyes.

They also provide essential fatty acids that the body cannot produce on its own. Here's a comprehensive look at healthy fats, including how to identify them on food labels, making it a pivotal section of the gestational diabetes food list.

Type of Fat	Sources	Benefits	What to Look for on Food Labels
Monounsaturated Fats	Avocados, olive oil, canola oil, nuts (almonds, peanuts, macadamia nuts), and seeds	Improves blood cholesterol levels, which can decrease the risk of heart disease. Aids in the development	Phrases like "high in monounsaturated fats" or specific mentions of olive oil, avocado oil, etc.

Type of Fat	Sources	Benefits	What to Look for on Food Labels
	(pumpkin, sesame).	of the baby's brain and nervous system.	
Polyunsaturated Fats	Walnuts, sunflower seeds, flaxseeds, chia seeds, fatty fish (salmon, mackerel, sardines), and soybean oil.	Contains omega-3 and omega-6 fatty acids, crucial for brain function and cell growth. Supports heart health and fetal development.	Look for terms like "rich in omega-3s" or "contains polyunsaturated fats." Specific mention of EPA and DHA (types of omega-3 fatty acids found in fish) is also a positive indicator.
Omega-3 Fatty Acids	Fatty fish (as above), flaxseeds, chia seeds,	Essential for brain development and function.	Labels may list specific omega-3 content, such as ALA (alpha-

Type of Fat	Sources	Benefits	What to Look for on Food Labels
	walnuts, and fortified eggs.	May reduce the risk of chronic diseases and improve heart health.	linolenic acid), EPA (eicosapentaenoic acid), and DHA (docosahexaenoic acid).
Saturated Fats (Limited Intake Recommended)	Coconut oil, butter, ghee, and fatty cuts of meat. While not "unhealthy" in moderation, they should be consumed less frequently.	Necessary in small amounts for hormone production and cellular membranes.	These will be listed simply as "saturated fat" on food labels. Aim for products with lower percentages of daily value (%DV) of saturated fats.

Tips for Reading Food Labels:

- **Total Fat:** Look for products with a higher proportion of their fats coming from monounsaturated and polyunsaturated fats rather than saturated fats.
- **Trans Fats:** Avoid trans fats completely if possible; they are harmful and can increase the risk of heart disease. Trans fats are often listed as "partially hydrogenated oils" on ingredients lists.
- **Serving Size:** Always check the serving size to ensure that the fat content fits within your dietary plan for managing gestational diabetes.

Incorporating Healthy Fats into Your Diet:

- **Cooking:** Use oils rich in monounsaturated and polyunsaturated fats for cooking and salad dressings.
- **Snacking:** opt for nuts and seeds as snacks instead of processed foods high in trans fats and saturated fats.
- **Balanced Intake:** While focusing on healthy fats, remember to balance them with adequate protein and fiber-rich carbohydrates to maintain blood sugar levels.

Understanding and selecting the right types of fats are crucial for managing gestational diabetes effectively. Healthy fats not only support fetal development but also contribute to the mother's well-being. By paying close attention to food labels and incorporating a variety of sources of beneficial fats, expectant mothers can navigate gestational diabetes with confidence, ensuring a healthy pregnancy and a strong start for their baby.

Dairy: Options and Alternatives

In managing gestational diabetes, dairy products and their alternatives play a versatile role, offering a rich source of calcium, protein, and other essential nutrients while needing careful consideration to balance blood sugar levels.

Here's a detailed table to guide expectant mothers in selecting dairy options and alternatives that fit within a gestational diabetes-friendly diet.

Dairy/Alternative	Key Nutrients	Considerations for Gestational Diabetes	Reading Food Labels
Low-fat Milk	Calcium, Vitamin D, Protein	Choose low-fat or skim versions to reduce saturated fat intake. Moderation is key due to natural sugars (lactose).	Look for added sugars in flavored milks. opt for unsweetened or plain versions. Check portion

Dairy/Alternative	Key Nutrients	Considerations for Gestational Diabetes	Reading Food Labels
Greek Yogurt	Protein, Calcium, Probiotics	High in protein and lower in sugar than regular yogurt. opt for plain versions and add fresh fruit for flavor.	sizes. Avoid products with added sugars or sweeteners. Verify live cultures for probiotic benefits. Be wary of added sodium.
Cottage Cheese	Protein, Calcium	A low-carbohydrate option that's versatile. Choose low-fat versions to reduce saturated fat.	Choose brands with lower sodium content.
Cheese	Calcium, Protein, Fat	opt for lower-fat versions like	Check for sodium and

Dairy/Alternative	Key Nutrients	Considerations for Gestational Diabetes	Reading Food Labels
		mozzarella or cottage cheese. Cheese is low in carbohydrates but can be high in fat and calories.	fat content. Aim for lower-fat and lower-sodium options.
Almond Milk	Vitamin E, Calcium (fortified), Vitamin D (fortified)	A low-carbohydrate alternative to cow's milk. Choose unsweetened varieties to avoid added sugars.	Ensure it's fortified with calcium and vitamin D. Avoid versions with added sugars or sweeteners.
Soy Milk	Protein, Vitamin D (fortified), Calcium (fortified)	Closest to cow's milk in protein content. opt for unsweetened versions.	Check fortification for calcium and vitamin D. Choose unsweetened

Dairy/Alternative	Key Nutrients	Considerations for Gestational Diabetes	Reading Food Labels
Oat Milk	Fiber, Vitamin D (fortified), Calcium (fortified)	Higher in carbohydrates than other plant-based options. Best consumed in moderation.	to minimize sugar intake. Look for unsweetened versions. Check fortification levels for calcium and vitamin D.
Coconut Milk (beverage)	Vitamin B12 (fortified), Vitamin D (fortified), Calcium (fortified)	Lower in protein and potentially higher in saturated fats. Use sparingly.	opt for unsweetened varieties. Check for fortification with vitamins and calcium.

Key Takeaways for Dairy and Alternatives in Gestational Diabetes:

- **Moderation and Balance**: While dairy and its alternatives can be part of a gestational diabetes diet, balancing carbohydrate intake and overall calories is crucial. Incorporating these products should not exceed recommended daily carbohydrate or calorie intakes.
- **Reading Labels**: Always read food labels for dairy and dairy alternatives. Key factors include added sugars, total carbohydrate content, fortification (particularly for plant-based options), and serving size. This ensures that the choice aligns with nutritional needs and gestational diabetes management goals.
- **Nutritional Value**: Choose products that offer the highest nutritional value, such as those high in protein and calcium and fortified with essential vitamins. This supports both maternal health and fetal development.
- **Personal Preference and Tolerance**: Individual preferences and dietary tolerances should guide choices. For example, some may prefer plant-based options due to lactose intolerance or ethical reasons, while others might lean towards traditional dairy for its protein and calcium content.

Incorporating the right mix of dairy or dairy alternatives into a diet for managing gestational diabetes can contribute to a balanced, nutrient-rich diet that supports both the mother's and baby's health. With careful selection and an eye on food labels, expectant mothers can navigate their choices confidently, ensuring they meet their nutritional needs without compromising blood glucose control.

Snacks: Healthy Choices to Keep You Going

In the context of managing gestational diabetes, snacks play a crucial role in maintaining steady blood glucose levels throughout the day. Choosing the right snacks can prevent spikes and dips in blood sugar, ensuring both mother and baby receive consistent energy and nutrition. Below is a detailed table highlighting healthy snack choices, their benefits, and what to look for on food labels to make informed decisions.

This guide is designed to be an integral part of a gestational diabetes food list, aiding in the selection of snacks that are not only safe but also beneficial.

Snack Option	Benefits for Gestational Diabetes	Key Nutrients	What to Look for on Food Labels
Nuts and Seeds	Provide healthy fats, proteins, and fiber which can help regulate blood sugar levels.	Protein, Fiber, Healthy Fats (Omega-3s), Magnesium, Zinc	Low sodium; no added sugars. Check for serving size to manage calorie

Snack Option	Benefits for Gestational Diabetes	Key Nutrients	What to Look for on Food Labels
			intake.
Greek Yogurt	High in protein and calcium, and can be paired with fruits or nuts for a balanced snack.	Protein, Calcium, Probiotics	Low-fat or non-fat options; no added sugars. Look for live cultures for digestive health.
Vegetable Sticks with Hummus	A low-calorie option that offers fiber and protein, helping to keep blood sugar levels stable.	Fiber, Protein, Healthy Fats, Vitamins A and C	Low sodium hummus; no added sugars or oils in hummus. Check for natural ingredients.
Whole Grain Crackers with	The combination of fiber from whole grains and protein from	Fiber, Protein, Calcium	Whole grains as the first ingredient; low in saturated fat.

Snack Option	Benefits for Gestational Diabetes	Key Nutrients	What to Look for on Food Labels
Cheese	cheese provides sustained energy.		Choose low-fat cheese.
Hard-Boiled Eggs	A protein-rich snack that can help maintain steady blood glucose levels.	Protein, Vitamin D, Choline	N/A (whole food). Choose organic or free-range eggs, if possible, for higher omega-3 content.
Sliced Apples with Almond Butter	Offers a good mix of carbohydrates, protein, and healthy fats for balanced blood sugar.	Fiber, Healthy Fats, Vitamin E, Magnesium	Low or no added sugars in almond butter. Look for short ingredient lists without fillers.

Snack Option	Benefits for Gestational Diabetes	Key Nutrients	What to Look for on Food Labels
Berries and Cottage Cheese	Berries provide antioxidants and fiber, while cottage cheese adds protein and calcium.	Antioxidants, Fiber, Protein, Calcium	Low-fat or non-fat cottage cheese; check berries for freshness or go for frozen without added sugars.
Chia Seed Pudding	Chia seeds are high in fiber and omega-3 fatty acids, which can support blood sugar management.	Omega-3 Fatty Acids, Fiber, Protein, Calcium	Homemade with controlled ingredients; for pre-made, look for no added sugars and low in calories.
Air-Popped Popcorn	A whole grain snack that's low in calories and high in fiber, providing a feeling of fullness.	Fiber, Antioxidants	No added butter or salt. Look for plain varieties that you can season at home with a pinch of

Snack Option	Benefits for Gestational Diabetes	Key Nutrients	What to Look for on Food Labels
Roasted Chickpeas	A crunchy, protein-rich snack that's also high in fiber.	Protein, Fiber, Iron, Magnesium	salt or herbs. Low sodium; no added oils. Look for simple ingredient lists or make at home for the best control over seasoning.

When managing gestational diabetes, understanding food labels is key to making healthy choices. Focus on snacks that are rich in fiber, protein, and healthy fats, while being low in added sugars and unhealthy fats. Monitoring portion sizes is also crucial, as even healthy foods can lead to excessive calorie intake if not properly portioned. Integrating these snacks into your daily diet can help manage blood sugar levels effectively, contributing to a healthier pregnancy.

Foods to Limit or Avoid

High Glycemic Index Fruits and Vegetables

In managing gestational diabetes, understanding the glycemic index (GI) of foods is crucial. The GI measures how quickly a food can raise blood sugar levels after eating. For individuals with gestational diabetes, focusing on foods with a low to moderate GI can help maintain stable blood glucose levels.

This is particularly important when it comes to fruits and vegetables, which, although packed with nutrients, can vary greatly in their glycemic impact. Below is a detailed table highlighting high glycemic index fruits and vegetables that are best limited or avoided in a gestational diabetes diet, along with reasons for their limitation.

High Glycemic Index Fruits and Vegetables	GI Range	Reasons to Limit or Avoid
Watermelon	72-80	Watermelon has a high GI, meaning it can cause a rapid increase in blood sugar levels.

High Glycemic Index Fruits and Vegetables	GI Range	Reasons to Limit or Avoid
		While nutritious, its consumption should be moderated.
Pineapple	66-76	Pineapple's high sugar content and GI can lead to quick spikes in glucose levels, making it less ideal for those managing gestational diabetes.
Mango	51-60	Despite its vitamin content, mangoes have a moderate to high GI, potentially raising blood sugar levels more than other fruits.
Potatoes (Boiled)	78-88	Boiled potatoes have a high GI, which can lead to quick rises in blood sugar. Alternatives like sweet potatoes have a lower GI and are more fiber-rich.
Parsnips	52-97	Parsnips can vary greatly in

High Glycemic Index Fruits and Vegetables	GI Range	Reasons to Limit or Avoid
		GI but often lean towards the higher end, making them a vegetable to limit for stable blood sugar management.
Pumpkin	75	Pumpkin has a high GI, which may contribute to rapid increases in glucose levels post-consumption.
Dates	42-62	Dates, while nutrient-dense, are high in sugars and can have a significant impact on blood sugar levels.
Instant Mashed Potatoes	85+	Instant mashed potatoes are processed and have a very high GI, leading to quick spikes in blood sugar levels.
Rutabagas	72	Rutabagas can quickly raise blood sugar due to their high GI, despite being a nutritious vegetable.
Corn Flakes	81	While not a fruit or

High Glycemic Index Fruits and Vegetables	GI Range	Reasons to Limit or Avoid
		vegetable, corn flakes are included to highlight the impact of processed grains, which often have a very high GI and are best avoided.

Why You Should Avoid High GI Fruits and Vegetables

1. **Rapid Blood Sugar Spikes**: High GI foods cause a quick rise in blood sugar levels, which can be hard to manage for individuals with gestational diabetes, potentially leading to hyperglycemia.
2. **Increased Insulin Demand**: Consuming foods that rapidly increase blood sugar levels can lead to a higher demand for insulin, which is already a concern in gestational diabetes.
3. **Risk of Gestational Complications**: Uncontrolled blood sugar levels can increase the risk of pregnancy complications, including the risk of developing type 2 diabetes post-pregnancy and larger birth weight for the baby.
4. **Nutrient Balance**: While fruits and vegetables are important for a balanced diet, focusing on those with a lower GI can

provide the necessary nutrients without the added risk of blood sugar spikes.

It's important to note that moderation and context are key. Pairing higher GI foods with those rich in fiber, protein, or healthy fats can mitigate their impact on blood sugar levels. Additionally, individual responses to different foods can vary, so monitoring blood sugar levels and consulting with a healthcare provider for personalized advice is recommended.

Processed and Junk Foods

Category	Processed and Junk Foods to Limit or Avoid	Why You Should Avoid
Sugary Snacks and Beverages	- Candy bars - Soda and sweetened beverages - Packaged sweets and pastries	- High in refined sugars which can spike blood glucose levels - Lack nutritional value and contribute to excessive weight gain - Can lead to an increased risk of gestational diabetes complications
Refined Grains	- White bread - Regular pasta - White rice - Packaged snacks made from refined flours	- Low in fiber, leading to rapid spikes in blood sugar - Nutrient-stripped compared to their whole grain counterparts - Can contribute to gestational weight gain beyond healthy recommendations
Processed Meats	- Sausages - Bacon - Deli meats	- Often high in sodium and preservatives, contributing to elevated blood pressure - May contain harmful additives like

Category	Processed and Junk Foods to Limit or Avoid	Why You Should Avoid
		nitrates and nitrites - Linked to increased risk of gestational diabetes when consumed in high amounts
Fast Foods	- Fried foods like French fries and chicken nuggets Burgers and pizza with high-fat content - High-calorie salads with creamy dressings	- Typically, high in trans fats and saturated fats, affecting heart health - Calorie-dense with little nutritional benefit, contributing to excessive weight gain - Often contain large amounts of sodium, risking water retention and hypertension
High-Fat Dairy and Cheese	- Full-fat milk - Cream - High-fat cheeses	- Saturated fats in high-fat dairy products can increase cholesterol levels - May contribute to weight gain if consumed in excess - Lower-fat dairy options provide calcium and protein without the added risks
Salty	- Chips - Pretzels -	- High sodium content can lead to

Category	Processed and Junk Foods to Limit or Avoid	Why You Should Avoid
Snacks	Packaged popcorn	increased blood pressure and edema (swelling) - Often contain unhealthy fats and additives - Provide little to no nutritional value and displace healthier snack options
Sweetened Breakfast Cereals	- Cereals with added sugars - Instant oatmeal packets with flavors	- High sugar content can cause quick spikes in blood sugar - Often low in fiber and protein, leading to hunger shortly after eating - Healthier options include unsweetened whole grain cereals and plain oats

Understanding the impact of processed and junk foods on gestational diabetes is crucial for managing the condition effectively. These foods are typically high in added sugars, unhealthy fats, and sodium, while offering little nutritional value. Consuming them can lead to rapid spikes in blood glucose levels, excessive weight gain, and an increased risk of pregnancy complications. By focusing on whole, nutrient-dense foods and minimizing the intake of processed options, expectant mothers can support their health and the health of their baby, maintaining stable blood sugar levels and promoting overall well-being during pregnancy.

Sugary Beverages and Sweets

Managing gestational diabetes involves careful monitoring of one's diet to maintain blood glucose levels within a healthy range. Sugary beverages and sweets are two categories that play a significant role in this management due to their potential to cause rapid spikes in blood sugar.

Below is a detailed table explaining these categories, why they should be avoided, and the effects they can have on both maternal and fetal health.

Category	Examples	Reasons to Avoid	Potential Effects
Sugary Beverages	- Soda - Fruit juices with added sugar - Energy drinks - Sweetened iced tea - Specialty coffees with added syrups and sugars	- High in simple sugars, leading to quick and significant increases in blood glucose levels. - Lack nutritional value, contributing empty calories without satiety. - Can lead to excessive weight gain	- Increased risk of gestational diabetes complications such as high birth weight and preterm birth. - Higher

Category	Examples	Reasons to Avoid	Potential Effects
		and increased insulin resistance.	likelihood of developing type 2 diabetes post-pregnancy for the mother. - Elevated risk of obesity and type 2 diabetes in children later in life.
Sweets	- Candy - Desserts (cakes, pies, pastries) - Sweetened yogurts - Ice cream - Chocolate (with high sugar content)	- Contain high amounts of refined sugars and unhealthy fats, leading to rapid blood sugar spikes. - Often high in calories, contributing to unnecessary weight gain. - Can displace more	- May exacerbate blood glucose management issues. - Increases risk of gestational weight gain and associated

Category	Examples	Reasons to Avoid	Potential Effects
		nutritious food choices, leading to deficiencies.	complications (e.g., preeclampsia, cesarean delivery). - Can negatively impact fetal development and long-term health outcomes for the child.

Key Takeaways:

- **Sugary Beverages and Sweets in Moderation**: While completely eliminating these items from one's diet might not be necessary, they should be consumed in moderation, and healthier alternatives should be considered.
- **Reading Labels**: Always read nutrition labels to check for added sugars even in products that might seem healthy, such as fruit juices or flavored yogurts.

- **Alternative Sweeteners**: While some might consider alternative sweeteners as a substitute, it's important to consult with a healthcare provider or a dietitian to understand the best choices, as some artificial sweeteners may have undesirable effects during pregnancy.
- **Hydration and Healthy Snacks**: Opting for water, unsweetened herbal teas, or milk for hydration and choosing whole fruits, nuts, or small portions of dark chocolate as snacks can satisfy sweet cravings healthily and nutritiously.

In conclusion, for those managing gestational diabetes, paying close attention to the consumption of sugary beverages and sweets is crucial. Making informed, health-conscious decisions about these foods can significantly impact the well-being of both mother and child, steering the pregnancy toward a healthier outcome for both.

Fatty Meats and High-Fat Dairy Products

Foods to Limit or Avoid	Reasons to Avoid	Impact on Gestational Diabetes
Fatty Meats	- High in saturated fats, which can contribute to increased cholesterol levels and heart disease risk. - Often contain higher levels of hormones and preservatives, which can impact overall health. - More difficult to digest, leading to discomfort and potentially impacting nutrient absorption.	- Can lead to elevated blood glucose levels indirectly by increasing insulin resistance. - May affect the hormonal balance necessary for managing gestational diabetes effectively. - Slower digestion can affect blood sugar management and lead to spikes or drops in glucose levels.
Examples: - Ribeye steak - Pork belly		

Foods to Limit or Avoid	Reasons to Avoid	Impact on Gestational Diabetes
- Sausages with high fat content - Lamb chops		
High-Fat Dairy Products	- Similar to fatty meats, they are high in saturated fats, affecting cardiovascular health. - Often calorie-dense, which can contribute to excessive weight gain during pregnancy. - Can displace other nutrient-dense foods from the diet due to their high satiety levels.	- Excessive intake can contribute to insulin resistance, complicating blood sugar control. - Weight management is crucial in gestational diabetes; excessive gain can worsen insulin resistance. - May lead to nutritional imbalances, affecting both mother's and baby's health.
Examples: - Cream - Full-fat		

Foods to Limit or Avoid	Reasons to Avoid	Impact on Gestational Diabetes
cheese		
- Whole milk		
- Butter		

In managing gestational diabetes, the focus is not only on controlling blood sugar levels but also on ensuring overall nutritional well-being. Fatty meats and high-fat dairy products, while permissible in small amounts, should be limited to maintain a balanced and healthful diet. The emphasis on moderation and selection of leaner protein sources, as well as low-fat dairy options, supports effective gestational diabetes management and promotes the health of both the expectant mother and the baby.

Alcohol and Caffeine

Substance	Reasons to Avoid	Impact on Gestational Diabetes	Recommended Guidelines
Alcohol	Alcohol consumption during pregnancy is strongly advised against due to its direct link to a range of developmental disorders and complications, such as fetal alcohol spectrum disorders (FASDs). Unlike nutrients and other substances, alcohol offers no benefit to fetal development and poses significant risks.	Alcohol can complicate the management of gestational diabetes by affecting blood sugar levels unpredictably. It can either increase or decrease blood glucose levels, making it harder to maintain control. Additionally, alcohol impairs liver function, affecting the liver's ability to release glucose, which can particularly	The safest approach during pregnancy is abstinence from alcohol. No amount of alcohol has been proven safe at any time during pregnancy. This aligns with guidelines from major health organizations worldwide.

Substance	Reasons to Avoid	Impact on Gestational Diabetes	Recommended Guidelines
		problematic for managing gestational diabetes.	
Caffeine	While not as universally advised against as alcohol, caffeine consumption during pregnancy is recommended to be limited. High levels of caffeine intake have been associated with low birth weight, preterm birth, and in some studies, increased risk of miscarriage. Caffeine is a stimulant that can increase heart rate	The relationship between caffeine and blood sugar levels is complex. Some research suggests that caffeine can influence insulin sensitivity, potentially making it more challenging to manage gestational diabetes. However, the effects can vary significantly from person to person.	Most health guidelines suggest limiting caffeine intake to less than 200 mg per day during pregnancy. This is roughly the amount in one 12-ounce cup of coffee. It's important to consider all sources of caffeine, including tea, soft drinks,

Substance	Reasons to Avoid	Impact on Gestational Diabetes	Recommended Guidelines
	and blood pressure, which requires moderation during pregnancy.		energy drinks, and chocolate, when tallying daily intake.

This table offers a concise overview of why alcohol and caffeine are substances to limit or avoid entirely during pregnancy, especially in the context of managing gestational diabetes. The overarching aim is to prioritize fetal health and ensure the mother's well-being, making informed choices about consumption critical. Adopting a cautious approach to these substances can significantly contribute to a healthy pregnancy outcome.

Reading Food Labels

Understanding Carbohydrate Counts

Understanding carbohydrate counts is foundational in managing gestational diabetes effectively. Carbohydrates directly impact blood sugar levels more significantly than fats and proteins, making it crucial for expectant mothers with gestational diabetes to become adept at reading food labels to manage their condition successfully. This skill enables them to make informed dietary choices, ensuring both their health and the health of their developing baby.

The Basics of Carbohydrates on Food Labels

Food labels provide essential information about the nutritional content of food items, including total carbohydrate content, which is listed in grams. This total includes all types of carbohydrates present in the food: sugars, starches, and dietary fiber.

1. **Total Carbohydrates**: This figure is your starting point. It tells you the total amount of carbohydrates in a single serving of the food product. Keeping track of your total carbohydrate intake is crucial in managing blood sugar levels.

2. **Dietary Fiber**: Found under the total carbohydrates, dietary fiber is a type of carbohydrate that the body can't fully digest. Unlike other carbs, fiber doesn't significantly raise blood sugar levels, so it can be subtracted from the total carbs when calculating your intake. High-fiber foods can help manage blood sugar peaks and are beneficial for overall digestive health.

3. **Sugars**: Also under the total carbohydrates, this number includes both added sugars and naturally occurring sugars (such as those in fruit and milk). Added sugars are more concerning for blood sugar management as they can cause rapid increases in blood sugar levels. Foods low in added sugars are preferable for managing gestational diabetes.

4. **Sugar Alcohols**: Sometimes used in sugar-free and Low-carb products, sugar alcohols can have a lesser impact on blood sugar levels compared to regular sugar. However, they can still affect blood sugar to some extent and may cause digestive discomfort if consumed in large amounts.

Why Understanding Carbohydrate Counts Is Important

For those managing gestational diabetes, understanding and controlling carbohydrate intake is vital. Carbohydrates are the primary energy source for both the mother and the baby but require careful management to avoid spikes in blood sugar levels. Learning to read food labels helps expectant mothers identify foods that fit within their carbohydrate budget for each meal and snack, enabling better blood sugar control.

Practical Tips for Reading Food Labels

- Pay Attention to Serving Size: The nutritional information provided is often for a specific serving size. Compare this to the amount you're actually consuming to accurately calculate your carbohydrate intake.
- Look Beyond "Net Carbs": Some products will advertise "net carbs," which subtract fiber and sometimes sugar alcohols from total carbs. While useful, it's essential to understand how each component (fiber, sugar, sugar alcohols) affects your body specifically, as individual responses can vary.

- Consider the Glycemic Index: Though not typically listed on food labels, being mindful of the glycemic index (GI) of foods can be helpful. Foods with a lower GI are generally better for managing blood sugar levels.
- Balance and Variety: Incorporating a variety of foods into your diet can help ensure you're getting a mix of slow-acting and fast-acting carbohydrates, along with necessary vitamins and minerals for both you and your baby.

For those navigating gestational diabetes, mastering the art of reading food labels is a critical tool in managing the condition. By understanding carbohydrate counts and their components, expectant mothers can make empowered dietary choices that support their health and the development of their baby. This knowledge, combined with guidance from healthcare providers, lays a solid foundation for healthy pregnancy outcomes.

Identifying Added Sugars

Reading food labels is a critical skill for managing gestational diabetes effectively, particularly when it comes to identifying added sugars. Added sugars are those not naturally present in foods but added during processing or preparation. They can significantly impact blood glucose levels, making it essential for expectant mothers with gestational diabetes to become adept at spotting them on food labels.

The first step in identifying added sugars is to look at the ingredient list. Added sugars can go by many names, making them somewhat tricky to recognize. Beyond the obvious terms like "sugar," "cane sugar," or "syrup," added sugars may also be listed as "high-fructose corn syrup," "dextrose," "fructose," "glucose," "maltose," "sucrose," "honey," "agave nectar," "molasses," and "maple syrup," among others. The variety of terms used underscores the importance of familiarizing oneself with these aliases to make informed decisions.

Moreover, the order in which ingredients are listed provides valuable insight. Ingredients are listed by quantity, from highest to lowest. If a form of sugar is listed among the first few ingredients, it indicates that the product contains a significant number of added sugars.

Nutrition facts labels are also instrumental in identifying added sugars. In the United States, food labels have undergone updates to include a line for "added sugars," both in grams and as a percentage of the Daily Value (DV). This change makes it easier to understand precisely how much sugar has been added to the product, beyond what naturally occurs in the food ingredients. For managing gestational diabetes, keeping added sugars to a minimum is crucial. The American Heart Association recommends that women limit their intake of added sugars to no more than 6 teaspoons (about 24 grams) per day. However, for those with gestational diabetes, even stricter vigilance may be warranted to maintain blood glucose levels within target ranges.

It's also worth noting that foods marketed as "healthy" or "natural" can still contain significant amounts of added sugars. Even products like granola bars, yogurt, and whole-grain cereals, often perceived as healthy choices, can be laden with added sugars. Thus, reading labels is essential, regardless of the health claims on packaging.

Beverages deserve special attention as they are a common source of added sugars. Sodas, fruit drinks, flavored coffees, and teas can contain high amounts of sugar that significantly affect blood glucose levels. Opting for water, unsweetened teas, or milk can be a better choice for managing gestational diabetes.

The ability to identify added sugars on food labels is paramount for those managing gestational diabetes. By carefully examining ingredient lists, understanding the various names for added sugars, and paying close attention to the nutrition facts label, expectant mothers can make informed choices that support their health and the health of their baby. Limiting intake of added sugars is not just about avoiding sweets; it's about scrutinizing packaged foods and beverages to ensure they align with gestational diabetes management goals. This level of diligence supports optimal pregnancy outcomes and sets the foundation for a healthy lifestyle beyond.

Recognizing Healthy Fats

Recognizing healthy fats on food labels is a crucial skill for anyone managing gestational diabetes, as the type of fat consumed can impact both maternal health and the development of the fetus. Fats are essential for fetal growth, brain development, and the absorption of fat-soluble vitamins, yet not all fats are created equal. Differentiating between healthy and unhealthy fats on food labels ensures that pregnant women can make informed dietary choices that support their gestational diabetes management and overall health.

When scanning food labels, the first step is to look at the total fat content, which is then broken down into saturated fats, trans fats, and sometimes, monounsaturated and polyunsaturated fats. For managing gestational diabetes and promoting heart health, the focus should be on minimizing intake of saturated and trans fats while emphasizing monounsaturated and polyunsaturated fats.

Saturated Fats are found in animal products like butter, cheese, red meat, and certain plant oils like palm and coconut oil. While they can be part of a balanced diet, excessive intake of saturated fats is linked to increased cholesterol levels and a higher risk of heart disease. Pregnant women should limit saturated fat to less than 10% of their total daily calories.

Trans Fats are the fats to avoid. They are often found in processed foods, baked goods, and fried foods. Trans fats raise bad cholesterol levels (LDL) and lower good cholesterol levels (HDL), increasing the risk of heart disease. Thankfully, due to regulatory changes, trans fats are less commonly found in foods, but it's still important to check labels for "partially hydrogenated oils," a source of trans fats.

Monounsaturated Fats and Polyunsaturated Fats are known as the healthy fats. Monounsaturated fats are present in olive oil, avocados, and nuts. These fats can help reduce bad cholesterol levels and are beneficial for heart health. Polyunsaturated fats include omega-3 and omega-6 fatty acids, found in fatty fish (like salmon and mackerel), flaxseeds, and walnuts. Omega-3 fatty acids are especially important during pregnancy as they support fetal brain and eye development.

Another key aspect of reading food labels for healthy fats is to check the serving size and the corresponding fat content to ensure appropriate portion control. This is particularly important for managing gestational diabetes, where maintaining a balanced intake of nutrients, including fats, can help regulate blood sugar levels.

In addition to recognizing the types of fats, it's also helpful to look for foods that are labeled as "low in saturated fat," "contains unsaturated fat," or "high in omega-3s." These labels can quickly guide you to healthier fat choices. However, it's still important to read the detailed nutritional information, as some products may be high in calories or contain added sugars, negating the benefits of healthy fats.

Lastly, integrating healthy fats into a gestational diabetes diet doesn't just involve reading labels but also making conscious food choices and preparing meals in ways that preserve the health benefits of these fats. For example, opting for baking or grilling over frying can help maintain the nutritional profile of fatty foods, particularly fish and poultry.

By understanding how to recognize healthy fats on food labels, pregnant women can make dietary choices that positively impact their gestational diabetes management and overall pregnancy health. This knowledge empowers them to select foods that will provide the best nutritional support for themselves and their developing babies.

Meal Planning and Preparation

Sample Meal Plans

Meal Type	Ingredients	How to Cook	Nutritional Information
Breakfast	Rolled oats, chia seeds, almond milk, fresh berries, a handful of nuts	Combine ½ cup rolled oats, 1 tablespoon chia seeds, and 1 cup almond milk in a bowl. Refrigerate overnight. In the morning, top with ½ cup fresh berries and a handful of nuts.	High in fiber and protein, low in sugar. Provides sustained energy and helps with blood sugar control.
Mid-Morning Snack	Greek yogurt, cinnamon, sliced apple	Mix 1 cup of Greek yogurt with ¼ teaspoon of cinnamon. Serve with a sliced	Rich in protein and calcium. Cinnamon can help control blood sugar

Meal Type	Ingredients	How to Cook	Nutritional Information
		medium apple on the side.	levels. The apple provides fiber.
Lunch	Mixed greens, grilled chicken breast, avocado, cherry tomatoes, olive oil, lemon juice	Grill a 4-ounce chicken breast and slice. Toss with 2 cups of mixed greens, ½ diced avocado, ½ cup cherry tomatoes. Dress with 1 tablespoon olive oil and 2 tablespoons lemon juice.	Balanced with lean protein, healthy fats, and low-carb vegetables. Aids in maintaining steady blood sugar levels.
Afternoon Snack	Carrot sticks, hummus	Slice carrots into sticks and serve with ¼ cup of hummus for dipping.	High in fiber and protein; hummus provides healthy fats.
Dinner	Quinoa, steamed	Bake a 4-ounce salmon fillet at	Offers a balance of complex carbs,

Meal Type	Ingredients	How to Cook	Nutritional Information
	broccoli, baked salmon, lemon, herbs	375°F for 15-20 minutes with lemon slices and herbs. Serve with ½ cup cooked quinoa and 1 cup steamed broccoli.	protein, omega-3 fatty acids, and essential nutrients.
Evening Snack	Cottage cheese, ground flaxseed, a few raspberries	Mix ½ cup of cottage cheese with 1 tablespoon of ground flaxseed. Top with a handful of raspberries.	High in protein and fiber. Flaxseeds provide omega-3 fatty acids.

This table provides a sample meal plan designed to cater to the needs of individuals managing gestational diabetes, emphasizing balanced macronutrients and sufficient fiber to regulate blood sugar levels throughout the day. Each meal is constructed to provide nutritional balance, with a focus on ingredients that support blood sugar management and overall health during pregnancy.

Shopping List Essentials

What to Buy	Food Label Considerations
Whole Grains (e.g., brown rice, quinoa, whole wheat pasta)	Look for the word "whole" as the first ingredient. Check for high fiber content (at least 3g per serving) and minimal added sugars.
Fresh Vegetables (especially non-starchy ones like leafy greens, bell peppers, broccoli)	Fresh vegetables don't come with labels, but when choosing packaged, go for those without added sauces or seasonings that may contain sugars and sodium.
Fresh Fruits (focus on low glycemic index options such as berries, apples, pears)	Similar to vegetables, fresh fruits don't have labels. For canned or packaged fruits, ensure they're in water or their own juice, not syrup.
Lean Proteins (chicken breast, turkey, fish, tofu, legumes)	For meats, check for the percentage of fat and opt for the leanest cuts. For canned legumes, look for low sodium or no salt added options.

What to Buy	Food Label Considerations
Healthy Fats (avocados, nuts, seeds, olive oil)	For oils, seek out those with a high content of monounsaturated and polyunsaturated fats. Nuts and seeds should be raw or dry roasted, without added oils or sugars.
Low-fat Dairy (Greek yogurt, cottage cheese, milk)	Choose products with low or no added sugars. For milk alternatives, ensure they're fortified with calcium and vitamin D and unsweetened.
Whole Grain Breads and Cereals	Check for whole grains as the first ingredient and a high fiber content. Avoid those with added sugars or honey in the first few ingredients.
Herbs and Spices (to add flavor without sodium or sugar)	opt for pure herbs and spices rather than mixes, which might contain added salts or sugars.
Water and Other Hydrating Fluids (unsweetened tea, sparkling water)	For flavored waters or teas, confirm there's no added sugar. Even "natural flavor" beverages should be consumed moderately.

This table encapsulates the essentials for a shopping list tailored for individuals managing gestational diabetes, offering guidance on selecting the most suitable food items and what to look for on food labels. The aim is to prioritize nutrient-dense foods that support blood sugar management while providing the necessary nutrients for both mother and baby's health. By focusing on whole foods and being vigilant about food labels, expectant mothers can make informed choices that promote well-being throughout the pregnancy.

Meal Prep Tips for Busy Expectant Mothers

Busy expectant mothers managing gestational diabetes face the unique challenge of needing to maintain a balanced, nutritious diet while juggling their often-hectic schedules. Meal prep is a crucial strategy for simplifying dietary management, ensuring that healthy choices are always at hand. Here are several meal prep tips tailored for gestational diabetes, designed to support blood sugar control and overall health.

First, planning is paramount. Dedicate a day each week to map out meals and snacks, focusing on a balance of proteins, complex carbohydrates, and healthy fats. Incorporating foods rich in fiber, such as vegetables and whole grains, can help slow the absorption of glucose into the bloodstream. Utilize a gestational diabetes food list to select ingredients that are nutritious and supportive of managing blood sugar levels.

Batch cooking is a time-saver that can make a significant difference. Preparing larger quantities of dishes like soups, stews, or casseroles allows for portions to be frozen and easily reheated. These meals can be designed to include a variety of vegetables, lean proteins, and whole grains, ensuring balanced nutrition in every bite.

Investing in the right storage containers can keep meals fresh and make portion control straightforward. Freezable, microwave-safe containers are ideal for storing pre-portioned meals. Labeling containers with the date and meal contents can help rotate meals efficiently, reducing waste and ensuring variety.

Snacking can be a challenge, but with preparation, it's easier to make healthy choices. Pre-portioned snacks, such as cut vegetables with hummus, a small handful of nuts, or Greek yogurt, can satisfy hunger between meals without spiking blood sugar levels. Keeping these ready-to-eat snacks on hand in the fridge or pantry can prevent reaching for less optimal choices.

Hydration is crucial for managing gestational diabetes, but busy schedules can make it easy to forget to drink enough water. Carrying a reusable water bottle can serve as a constant reminder to stay hydrated. Infusing water with slices of fruit or cucumber can add a refreshing twist, making it more appealing to drink throughout the day.

Simplify breakfast choices by preparing ahead. Overnight oats, chia seed puddings, or egg muffins can be made in batches and offer a quick, nutritious start to the day. Incorporating protein and fiber in breakfast options can help stabilize morning blood sugar levels.

When it comes to vegetables, roasting or steaming a week's worth in one go can save time. These can then be quickly added to salads, omelets, or grain bowls throughout the week, ensuring that meals are nutrient-dense and balanced.

Don't overlook the power of a well-stocked pantry. Having gestational diabetes-friendly staples on hand, such as whole grain pasta, quinoa, tinned legumes, nuts, seeds, and low-sugar sauces can make throwing together a healthy meal much quicker and easier.

Lastly, seeking support from family members or friends can make meal prep less daunting. Sharing the responsibility can not only lighten the load but also make the process more enjoyable. Plus, it offers a wonderful opportunity to educate loved ones about the dietary needs of gestational diabetes, making them more equipped to offer support.

By incorporating these meal prep tips into their routine, busy expectant mothers can navigate the challenges of gestational diabetes with confidence, ensuring they and their babies remain healthy and well-nourished throughout the pregnancy.

Eating Out and Social Events

Tips for Restaurant Dining

Navigating restaurant dining can be challenging for individuals managing gestational diabetes, but with a few strategic tips, it's entirely possible to enjoy eating out while keeping blood sugar levels in check. These strategies revolve around making informed food choices, understanding how dishes are prepared, and knowing how to request modifications that align with a gestational diabetes-friendly diet.

Start by researching restaurants ahead of time. Many establishments now offer their menus online, allowing you to preview options and decide on a few diabetes-friendly choices before arriving. Look for dishes that emphasize lean proteins, whole grains, and plenty of vegetables, which can help stabilize blood sugar levels. Salads with grilled chicken or fish, stir-fries loaded with vegetables, and entrees that feature lean cuts of meat are usually good choices.

When ordering, don't hesitate to ask questions about the menu. Inquire about the preparation methods of dishes to avoid those that are fried or cooked in excessive amounts of oil or butter. Instead, opt for meals that are steamed, grilled, baked, or roasted. These cooking techniques minimize added fats, helping you manage your calorie and fat intake better.

Request substitutions where necessary. Most restaurants are willing to accommodate dietary requests, such as substituting a side of fries or mashed potatoes with a garden salad or extra vegetables. If a dish comes with a sauce or dressing, ask for it on the side so you can control the amount you consume. This is particularly important for dressings and sauces that may be high in sugar or fat.

Be mindful of portion sizes, which are often larger in restaurants than at home. Consider ordering a starter as your main course or sharing a larger entree with a dining companion. Another strategy is to ask for half of your meal to be boxed up before it's brought to the table, ensuring you don't overeat.

Pay attention to carbohydrate intake, especially from sources that can spike blood sugar levels quickly. Limit or avoid dishes that include large amounts of pasta, white rice, and bread. If you're craving something starchy, look for options like quinoa, brown rice, or sweet potatoes, which have a lower glycemic index and provide more nutritional value.

Beverage choices also matter when dining out. Water, unsweetened iced tea, or sparkling water with a slice of lemon are preferable to sugary drinks, fruit juices, or alcoholic beverages, which can interfere with blood sugar management.

Finally, enjoy your meal mindfully. Eating slowly and savoring each bite can not only enhance your dining experience but also help you recognize when you're full, preventing overeating.

With these tips, restaurant dining can be a pleasurable experience that fits seamlessly into the management of gestational diabetes. By making informed choices, asking for modifications, and staying mindful of portion sizes and carbohydrate intake, you can maintain control over your blood sugar levels while enjoying the social and culinary pleasures of eating out.

Navigating Social Gatherings

Navigating social gatherings while managing gestational diabetes can pose a challenge, given the array of tempting foods and the desire to participate fully in celebrations. However, with a bit of planning and strategy, it's entirely possible to enjoy these events while keeping blood sugar levels in check. The key is preparation, understanding the gestational diabetes food list, and making informed choices about what to eat and drink.

One effective strategy is eating a small, balanced meal or snack before heading to an event. This can help stabilize blood sugar levels and reduce the temptation to indulge in high-carbohydrate or sugary foods. Including a good mix of protein, fiber, and healthy fats can keep you feeling fuller longer, making it easier to pass on less healthy options.

When at the event, first survey the entire spread of foods before making any selections. Look for items that fit within the gestational diabetes food list such as vegetables, fruits with a low glycemic index, lean proteins, and whole grains. These choices will not only nourish but also help maintain steady blood glucose levels. If possible, opt for grilled or baked dishes over fried options and choose sauces and dressings on the side to better control intake.

Portion control is another crucial aspect of managing gestational diabetes at social events. Even healthy foods can lead to high blood sugar levels if consumed in large quantities. Using a smaller plate can help manage portion sizes, and filling half the plate with vegetables before adding proteins or carbohydrates can keep portions in check.

Don't hesitate to bring your own dish to share. This ensures there will be at least one gestational diabetes-friendly option available, and hosts often appreciate the gesture. Choose a recipe that is both delicious and meets your dietary needs, so you feel included in the feast without compromising your health.

Beverage choices are equally important. Water, seltzer, and unsweetened iced tea are excellent choices. If you want something with a bit more flavor, consider adding a slice of lemon or lime to water. Steer clear of sugary drinks and alcohol, as they can quickly elevate blood sugar levels and offer no nutritional value.

Conversation and companionship are just as much a part of social gatherings as food. Focusing on the company rather than the cuisine can divert attention from eating and enhance the enjoyment of the event. Engaging in conversations, participating in activities or games, and enjoying the moment can shift the focus away from food.

Lastly, monitor your blood sugar levels before and after the event to understand how different foods and the amount of activity affect you. This feedback can be invaluable for future events, helping to refine strategies for managing gestational diabetes in social settings.

Attending social gatherings while managing gestational diabetes requires a balance of preparation, mindful eating, and focusing on the joy of the occasion beyond just the food. By making informed choices, staying hydrated, and enjoying the company of friends and family, it's possible to navigate these events successfully without compromising health goals.

Alcohol Alternatives and Mocktails

Navigating social events and dining out can be challenging for those managing gestational diabetes, especially when it comes to finding suitable drink options that align with dietary guidelines. With alcohol off the table during pregnancy, mocktails and alcohol-free alternatives present a delightful and safe way to enjoy a festive beverage without compromising health or blood sugar levels. These alternatives are not only safer for expectant mothers but can also be nutritious, adding a fun twist to hydration without the empty calories and sugar spikes associated with traditional alcoholic beverages.

When considering mocktails and alcohol-free alternatives, the key is to focus on ingredients that are low in sugars and high in flavor. Sparkling water serves as an excellent base for many mocktails, offering a fizzy satisfaction without added sugars or calories. Adding slices of fruits like lemons, limes, oranges, or even cucumbers can infuse natural flavors without significantly impacting blood sugar levels. For a touch of sweetness, opting for natural sweeteners like stevia or a small amount of agave syrup can provide the desired taste without the blood sugar rollercoaster that comes with refined sugars.

Herbs and spices also play a significant role in elevating the taste of mocktails. Mint, basil, and rosemary can add a fresh and aromatic dimension to drinks, while ginger can provide a zesty kick with the added benefit of aiding digestion, which can be particularly useful during pregnancy. The infusion of such ingredients not only enhances flavor but also incorporates antioxidants and nutrients beneficial to both maternal and fetal health.

Creating mocktails with a blend of 100% fruit juices diluted with sparkling water is another strategy for managing sugar intake while indulging in a flavorful drink. For example, mixing a quarter cup of cranberry juice with three-quarters cup of sparkling water and adding a squeeze of lime provides a festive beverage with a fraction of the sugar content of a standard cocktail or soft drink. It's important to always check the labels when choosing fruit juices, opting for those without added sugars or sweeteners to ensure the drink remains gestational diabetes-friendly.

For those eating out or attending social events, requesting custom-made mocktails with specific instructions can help maintain dietary control. Asking for drinks to be made without syrup, substituting soda water for tonic water, and specifying the type of sweetener and its quantity can make a significant difference in managing glucose levels. Additionally, being open to trying different herbal teas, both hot and iced, can offer a comforting or refreshing alternative that fits well within the parameters of a gestational diabetes diet.

Experimenting with alcohol alternatives and mocktails not only adheres to the dietary needs of managing gestational diabetes but also enriches the social and dining experience during pregnancy. These alternatives emphasize the opportunity to enjoy a wide array of flavors and ingredients that contribute to hydration and nutrition, turning the limitation on alcohol into an avenue for culinary creativity and healthful enjoyment. With thoughtful selection and preparation, mocktails can offer a delightful complement to the gestational diabetes food list, ensuring that social gatherings remain a source of pleasure and celebration.

Monitoring Blood Sugar Levels

The Importance of Monitoring

Monitoring blood sugar levels is a critical component of managing gestational diabetes, a condition that affects a significant number of pregnancies. This careful monitoring enables expecting mothers to understand how their bodies react to different foods, activities, and stress levels, providing insights that are essential for keeping both maternal and fetal health optimized.

For those navigating gestational diabetes, the food list becomes an invaluable tool, guiding dietary choices to ensure blood glucose levels remain within target ranges. Each individual's response to certain foods can vary, making it crucial to track blood sugar responses to specific dietary patterns. This personalized feedback loop allows for adjustments in meal planning and snacking, ensuring that the consumption of carbohydrates is balanced throughout the day to prevent spikes in blood sugar levels.

Moreover, monitoring blood sugar helps in identifying the effectiveness of dietary changes over time. By keeping a detailed record, expectant mothers, in collaboration with their healthcare providers, can discern patterns and make informed decisions about their diet. For instance, if consistently high readings are noted after meals containing certain fruits or grains, these items may be adjusted or replaced with alternatives that have a lesser impact on blood glucose.

Beyond dietary management, monitoring blood sugar levels plays a pivotal role in determining the need for medication or insulin. While diet and exercise are the first lines of defense in managing gestational diabetes, some cases may require additional interventions. Regular monitoring helps healthcare providers to make timely decisions regarding the introduction or adjustment of medication, tailored to the individual's needs.

The frequency of monitoring is another critical aspect. Generally, it's recommended to test blood sugar levels four times a day – fasting (upon waking) and after each main meal (postprandial). This regimen offers a comprehensive view of how well gestational diabetes is being managed and how the body is handling the intake of carbohydrates throughout the day.

Importantly, the process of monitoring and adjusting the diet based on blood sugar readings empowers women with gestational diabetes. It provides a sense of control and active participation in their health care and the well-being of their baby. This proactive approach can also mitigate the risk of pregnancy complications associated with gestational diabetes, such as preterm birth, excessive birth weight, and the development of type 2 diabetes in later life for both mother and child.

The synergy between a carefully curated gestational diabetes food list and diligent monitoring of blood sugar levels cannot be overstated. This combination is foundational in managing gestational diabetes effectively, ensuring a healthy pregnancy outcome. Through monitoring, expectant mothers gain invaluable insights into how their dietary choices influence their blood sugar levels, allowing for precise adjustments that safeguard their health and that of their developing baby.

How Food Affects Blood Sugar

Understanding how food affects blood sugar is fundamental in managing gestational diabetes. The body converts carbohydrates from food into glucose, which enters the bloodstream, raising blood sugar levels. This increase triggers the pancreas to release insulin, allowing glucose to move from the blood into the body's cells for energy. However, during pregnancy, hormonal changes can make the body's cells less responsive to insulin, a condition known as insulin resistance. This can lead to elevated blood sugar levels, necessitating careful monitoring and management, especially with a gestational diabetes diagnosis.

Carbohydrates have the most significant impact on blood sugar levels. Not all carbs are created equal; their effect on blood sugar can vary widely depending on the type of carbohydrate consumed. Foods high in refined sugars and starches, such as white bread, pastries, and sweets, are quickly broken down into glucose, leading to rapid spikes in blood sugar. Conversely, complex carbohydrates, found in whole grains, vegetables, and legumes, are digested more slowly, resulting in a gradual, more manageable increase in blood sugar.

Fiber, a type of carbohydrate that the body can't digest, plays a crucial role in moderating blood sugar levels. High-fiber foods slow down the digestion of other carbohydrates, which helps prevent sudden spikes in blood sugar. This makes high-fiber foods an essential component of a gestational diabetes diet.

Protein and fats also influence blood sugar, though to a lesser extent than carbohydrates. When consumed with carbohydrates, protein and fats can slow down the absorption of sugar into the bloodstream, helping to keep blood sugar levels stable. However, it's important to choose healthy sources of these macronutrients, such as lean meats, fish, nuts, seeds, and vegetable oils, to avoid additional health risks, such as high cholesterol or heart disease.

Glycemic index (GI) and glycemic load (GL) are useful tools in understanding how different foods affect blood sugar levels. The GI measures how quickly a food raises blood sugar levels compared to pure glucose, while the GL takes into account the amount of carbohydrate in a serving of the food as well as how quickly it raises blood sugar levels. Foods with a low GI or GL are preferable for managing gestational diabetes as they lead to more gradual increases in blood sugar.

Monitoring blood sugar levels is crucial for women with gestational diabetes to understand how their bodies respond to different foods and to manage their condition effectively. This typically involves checking blood sugar levels at various times throughout the day, such as fasting, before meals, and one to two hours after eating. Keeping a food diary can also be helpful, allowing for tracking of what was eaten and how it affected blood sugar levels. This information can be used to adjust meal plans and food choices to better control gestational diabetes.

Ultimately, managing gestational diabetes through diet focuses on balancing the intake of carbohydrates, proteins, and fats, choosing foods that contribute to stable blood sugar levels, and avoiding or limiting foods that can cause spikes. By understanding how food affects blood sugar and monitoring their blood sugar levels, pregnant women can take significant steps toward maintaining their health and ensuring the well-being of their babies.

Adjusting Your Diet Based on Blood Sugar Readings

Monitoring blood sugar levels is a crucial component of managing gestational diabetes, providing immediate feedback on how different foods and meals impact glucose levels. This dynamic process allows for a tailored approach to diet, ensuring both maternal and fetal health throughout pregnancy. By understanding the relationship between food intake and blood sugar readings, expectant mothers can make informed adjustments to their diet, optimizing their gestational diabetes food list for better glucose control.

Regular monitoring can reveal patterns in blood sugar fluctuations, highlighting specific foods or meals that may cause spikes or drops in glucose levels. This insight enables a personalized dietary strategy, focusing on maintaining a balance of nutrients while avoiding or modifying the intake of foods that adversely affect blood sugar control.

Incorporating a wide variety of whole foods rich in fiber, such as vegetables, whole grains, and legumes, can help moderate blood sugar levels. These foods slow the absorption of glucose into the bloodstream, providing a steady energy release and preventing sharp spikes in blood sugar. By closely observing how these foods influence individual blood sugar readings, adjustments can be made to portion sizes and meal composition to ensure optimal glycemic control.

Protein and healthy fats are also key components of a gestational diabetes-friendly diet, contributing to satiety and helping to minimize blood sugar spikes. Lean protein sources like chicken, fish, tofu, and legumes, alongside healthy fats from avocados, nuts, and seeds, can be incorporated based on personal blood sugar responses. Tailoring the ratio of macronutrients in meals and snacks according to blood sugar readings allows for a flexible and effective dietary plan.

Moreover, understanding the glycemic index of fruits and choosing those with a lower index can aid in fine-tuning sugar intake. Pairing carbohydrates with proteins or fats can further mitigate rapid increases in glucose levels, a strategy that can be refined through regular monitoring.

Meal timing and frequency also play a significant role in managing gestational diabetes. Eating smaller, more frequent meals can help maintain steady blood sugar levels throughout the day. Blood sugar readings can guide the adjustment of meal schedules, ensuring that glucose levels remain within target ranges without prolonged periods of fasting.

Hydration, often overlooked, is vital in managing blood sugar. Water does not raise blood sugar levels and can help in the metabolism of glucose. Monitoring can help identify if inadequate hydration correlates with higher blood sugar levels, prompting an increase in fluid intake.

Lastly, physical activity, in conjunction with diet, is essential for blood sugar management. Monitoring blood sugar before and after exercise can help in understanding its effects on glucose levels, allowing for dietary adjustments to accommodate increased energy expenditure or to prevent hypoglycemia.

In essence, adjusting one's diet based on blood sugar readings is an ongoing process of refinement and personalization. This approach not only aids in achieving better glycemic control but also supports a healthier pregnancy overall. The key lies in the willingness to observe, adapt, and modify dietary choices and lifestyle habits as needed, based on the feedback provided by regular blood sugar monitoring. This proactive engagement with one's health empowers expectant mothers to navigate gestational diabetes with confidence and resilience, ensuring the well-being of both mother and baby.

Exercise and Physical Activity

Safe Exercises During Pregnancy

Maintaining an active lifestyle during pregnancy, especially when managing gestational diabetes, plays a crucial role in promoting maternal health and fetal development. Exercise can help regulate blood sugar levels, reduce the risk of gestational diabetes becoming type 2 diabetes postpartum, and aid in managing weight gain throughout pregnancy. For those navigating the complexities of gestational diabetes, coupling a balanced diet from a carefully selected food list with safe exercises can optimize health outcomes for both the mother and baby.

Walking is one of the most recommended forms of exercise for pregnant women, offering a low-impact way to stay active. It doesn't require any special equipment other than a pair of supportive shoes, making it an accessible option for most. Walking helps improve cardiovascular health without putting too much strain on the knees and ankles, areas that can become more vulnerable during pregnancy due to natural increases in body weight and shifts in the center of gravity.

Prenatal yoga is another excellent option, known for its gentle stretches and stress-reducing benefits. It focuses on breathing and moving at a peaceful rhythm, which can be particularly beneficial for emotional well-being. Prenatal yoga classes are designed to accommodate the changing pregnant body and focus on poses that enhance flexibility, strength, and circulation, all while promoting relaxation and a deeper connection between mother and baby.

Swimming and water aerobics stand out as ideal exercises for gestational diabetes management. The buoyancy of water reduces the stress on weight-bearing joints and helps prevent overheating, making it a safe choice throughout all trimesters of pregnancy. These water-based activities can boost heart health, ease back pain, and improve muscle tone without the risk of injury.

Stationary cycling is another safe exercise during pregnancy, providing a good cardiovascular workout with minimal risk of falling. As balance can become an issue in later stages of pregnancy, stationary bikes offer a stable platform for a heart-healthy workout that can easily be adjusted for intensity and duration.

Low-impact aerobics classes, specifically designed for pregnant women, are beneficial for maintaining fitness in a controlled environment. These classes avoid high-impact moves, deep backbends, and jumps, focusing instead on maintaining heart rate at a safe level. They often include strength training components, using light weights or body weight to help maintain muscle tone and support posture.

Strength training exercises, when done correctly and with moderation in mind, can be particularly beneficial. Focusing on major muscle groups and avoiding heavy weights can help with posture, decrease common pregnancy pains, and enhance stamina needed for labor and delivery. It's important to avoid exercises that involve lying flat on the back or standing still for long periods, as these positions can restrict blood flow.

Regardless of the type of exercise chosen, the key is to listen to the body and adjust the activity level accordingly. Staying hydrated, avoiding overheating, and consuming a balanced diet rich in nutrients from the gestational diabetes food list will support exercise efforts, ensuring that blood sugar levels are managed effectively. It's also crucial to consult with a healthcare provider before starting any new exercise regimen during pregnancy, especially when managing gestational diabetes, to ensure all activities are safe for the mother's and baby's health.

Incorporating safe exercises into a daily routine can significantly contribute to a healthy pregnancy, complementing dietary measures taken to manage gestational diabetes. This holistic approach not only aids in immediate blood sugar control but also sets a foundation for long-term health and well-being.

The Impact of Physical Activity on Gestational Diabetes

Physical activity plays a crucial role in managing gestational diabetes, offering a synergistic effect when combined with a carefully curated food list. Exercise during pregnancy not only helps in controlling blood glucose levels but also contributes to overall health, improves mood, and reduces pregnancy-related discomforts.

Regular physical activity enhances insulin sensitivity, which means the body can use insulin more efficiently, reducing blood glucose levels. This is particularly beneficial for women with gestational diabetes, as their bodies struggle with insulin resistance. By incorporating exercise into daily routines, expectant mothers can better manage their blood glucose levels, minimizing the need for medication and reducing the risk of complications during pregnancy and delivery.

Moderate-intensity activities, such as brisk walking, swimming, or prenatal yoga, are generally recommended for pregnant women. These activities are effective in keeping blood sugar levels in check without placing undue stress on the body. It's important to engage in these activities most days of the week, aiming for at least 150 minutes of moderate-intensity exercise spread throughout the week.

The timing of exercise can also play a pivotal role in managing gestational diabetes. Engaging in physical activity shortly after meals can take advantage of the natural rise in blood glucose levels that occurs after eating, using this glucose as energy for the exercise. This helps in lowering postprandial (after-meal) blood glucose levels, a key factor in managing gestational diabetes.

Moreover, physical activity influences the body's need for insulin and can alter how it utilizes nutrients from food. For this reason, coordinating the gestational diabetes food list with exercise routines is essential. Consuming a balanced diet rich in fiber, lean proteins, and healthy fats provides the necessary energy for physical activity while aiding in steady blood glucose levels. It's beneficial to include a small, balanced snack before exercising to prevent hypoglycemia, especially if exercising for longer periods or at higher intensities.

Pregnant women with gestational diabetes should consult their healthcare provider before starting any exercise regimen. This ensures that the chosen activities are safe and appropriately matched to their individual health profile and pregnancy progression. Adjustments to diet and possibly medication dosages may be needed to accommodate increased physical activity.

Beyond managing gestational diabetes, physical activity during pregnancy has been linked to a shorter labor, reduced risk of Cesarean section, quicker postpartum recovery, and a lower likelihood of developing type 2 diabetes in the future. It also sets a foundation for a healthy lifestyle after delivery, benefiting the mother and her child in the long term.

Integrating physical activity with a gestational diabetes-friendly diet creates a comprehensive approach to managing blood glucose levels during pregnancy. This balanced strategy not only aids in controlling gestational diabetes but also supports overall health, ensuring a more comfortable and healthy pregnancy for both mother and baby.

Conclusion

In wrapping up the exploration of managing gestational diabetes through dietary choices, it becomes evident that a well-considered food list serves as a powerful tool in navigating this condition. The journey through understanding the role of macronutrients, the critical importance of micronutrients, and the considerations around substances like alcohol and caffeine, alongside the impact of physical activity, underscores a holistic approach to health during pregnancy.

The gestational diabetes food list is not merely a set of restrictions; it's a guide towards optimal health for both the mother and her developing baby. By focusing on whole grains, lean proteins, healthy fats, and a colorful array of fruits and vegetables, expectant mothers can manage their blood glucose levels more effectively. This approach not only mitigates the risks associated with gestational diabetes but also supports overall well-being.

Moreover, the emphasis on hydration, careful consideration of caffeine intake, and the avoidance of alcohol highlights the nuanced aspects of dietary management that can have significant impacts on blood glucose control and pregnancy outcomes. Coupling these dietary strategies with regular, moderate physical activity further enhances insulin sensitivity and glucose management, offering a robust defense against the challenges posed by gestational diabetes.

This comprehensive strategy does more than manage gestational diabetes; it sets the stage for a healthy lifestyle that can continue beyond pregnancy. It educates and empowers women to make informed choices about their health and the health of their babies. By taking control of their diet and incorporating physical activity into their routine, expectant mothers can not only navigate gestational diabetes more effectively but also lay a foundation for a healthy future for themselves and their families.

Ultimately, managing gestational diabetes with a thoughtful food list and lifestyle adjustments is about more than controlling blood sugar levels; it's about embracing a healthy pregnancy journey. It serves as a reminder that through informed choices and proactive management, expectant mothers can overcome the challenges of gestational diabetes, ensuring the best possible start for their babies and a healthier future for their families.

www.ingramcontent.com/pod-product-compliance
Lightning Source LLC
Chambersburg PA
CBHW050306230526
45471CB00005B/2055